THIS BOOK BELONGS TO:

CONTACT INFORMATION	
NAME:	
ADDRESS:	
PHONE:	

EMERGENCY CONTACT	
NAME:	
ADDRESS:	
PHONE:	

DEDICATION

This Diabetes Log Book is dedicated to all the people who want to track and collect data to keep their diabetes under control. Staying organized will help you share valuable information with your health care providers.

You are my inspiration for producing this book and I'm honored to be a part of your record-keeping and ongoing health care.

How to Use this Book

This Diabetes Log Book will help guide you by accurately recording blood glucose levels throughout the day.

Here are examples of tracking and prompts for you to fill in and write the details of your food intake, blood sugar readings, and physical activity:

1. Weekly Diabetes Log - Fill in readings for each day of the week.

2. Daily Log - Monday through Friday- record daily readings for blood sugar, insulin dose, grams of carbs, and physical activity.

3. Daily Meals - Log readings (pre and post) for each meal: breakfast, lunch, dinner, snacks, and bedtime.

4. Notes - A place to write daily information: medication, exercise, blood pressure, etc.

Weekly Diabetes Log

WEEK OF:		BREAKFAST		LUNCH		DINNER		SNACK #1		SNACK #2		BEDTIME	
		PRE	POST	PRE	POST	PRE	POST	PRE	POST	PRE	POST	PRE	POST
MONDAY	BLOOD SUGAR												
	INSULIN DOSE												
	GRAMS OF CARBS												
	PHYS. ACTIVITY												
TUESDAY	BLOOD SUGAR												
	INSULIN DOSE												
	GRAMS OF CARBS												
	PHYS. ACTIVITY												
WEDNESDAY	BLOOD SUGAR												
	INSULIN DOSE												
	GRAMS OF CARBS												
	PHYS. ACTIVITY												
THURSDAY	BLOOD SUGAR												
	INSULIN DOSE												
	GRAMS OF CARBS												
	PHYS. ACTIVITY												
FRIDAY	BLOOD SUGAR												
	INSULIN DOSE												
	GRAMS OF CARBS												
	PHYS. ACTIVITY												
SATURDAY	BLOOD SUGAR												
	INSULIN DOSE												
	GRAMS OF CARBS												
	PHYS. ACTIVITY												

Weekly Diabetes Log Book

NOTES

MONDAY

TUESDAY

WEDNESDAY

THURSDAY

FRIDAY

SATURDAY

Weekly Diabetes Log

WEEK OF:		BREAKFAST		LUNCH		DINNER		SNACK #1		SNACK #2		BEDTIME	
		PRE	POST	PRE	POST	PRE	POST	PRE	POST	PRE	POST	PRE	POST
MONDAY	BLOOD SUGAR												
	INSULIN DOSE												
	GRAMS OF CARBS												
	PHYS. ACTIVITY												
TUESDAY	BLOOD SUGAR												
	INSULIN DOSE												
	GRAMS OF CARBS												
	PHYS. ACTIVITY												
WEDNESDAY	BLOOD SUGAR												
	INSULIN DOSE												
	GRAMS OF CARBS												
	PHYS. ACTIVITY												
THURSDAY	BLOOD SUGAR												
	INSULIN DOSE												
	GRAMS OF CARBS												
	PHYS. ACTIVITY												
FRIDAY	BLOOD SUGAR												
	INSULIN DOSE												
	GRAMS OF CARBS												
	PHYS. ACTIVITY												
SATURDAY	BLOOD SUGAR												
	INSULIN DOSE												
	GRAMS OF CARBS												
	PHYS. ACTIVITY												

Weekly Diabetes Log Book

NOTES

MONDAY

TUESDAY

WEDNESDAY

THURSDAY

FRIDAY

SATURDAY

Weekly Diabetes Log

WEEK OF:		BREAKFAST		LUNCH		DINNER		SNACK #1		SNACK #2		BEDTIME	
		PRE	POST	PRE	POST	PRE	POST	PRE	POST	PRE	POST	PRE	POST
MONDAY	BLOOD SUGAR												
	INSULIN DOSE												
	GRAMS OF CARBS												
	PHYS. ACTIVITY												
TUESDAY	BLOOD SUGAR												
	INSULIN DOSE												
	GRAMS OF CARBS												
	PHYS. ACTIVITY												
WEDNESDAY	BLOOD SUGAR												
	INSULIN DOSE												
	GRAMS OF CARBS												
	PHYS. ACTIVITY												
THURSDAY	BLOOD SUGAR												
	INSULIN DOSE												
	GRAMS OF CARBS												
	PHYS. ACTIVITY												
FRIDAY	BLOOD SUGAR												
	INSULIN DOSE												
	GRAMS OF CARBS												
	PHYS. ACTIVITY												
SATURDAY	BLOOD SUGAR												
	INSULIN DOSE												
	GRAMS OF CARBS												
	PHYS. ACTIVITY												

Weekly Diabetes Log Book

NOTES

MONDAY

TUESDAY

WEDNESDAY

THURSDAY

FRIDAY

SATURDAY

Weekly Diabetes Log

WEEK OF:		BREAKFAST		LUNCH		DINNER		SNACK #1		SNACK #2		BEDTIME	
		PRE	POST	PRE	POST	PRE	POST	PRE	POST	PRE	POST	PRE	POST
MONDAY	BLOOD SUGAR												
	INSULIN DOSE												
	GRAMS OF CARBS												
	PHYS. ACTIVITY												
TUESDAY	BLOOD SUGAR												
	INSULIN DOSE												
	GRAMS OF CARBS												
	PHYS. ACTIVITY												
WEDNESDAY	BLOOD SUGAR												
	INSULIN DOSE												
	GRAMS OF CARBS												
	PHYS. ACTIVITY												
THURSDAY	BLOOD SUGAR												
	INSULIN DOSE												
	GRAMS OF CARBS												
	PHYS. ACTIVITY												
FRIDAY	BLOOD SUGAR												
	INSULIN DOSE												
	GRAMS OF CARBS												
	PHYS. ACTIVITY												
SATURDAY	BLOOD SUGAR												
	INSULIN DOSE												
	GRAMS OF CARBS												
	PHYS. ACTIVITY												

Weekly Diabetes Log Book

NOTES

MONDAY

TUESDAY

WEDNESDAY

THURSDAY

FRIDAY

SATURDAY

Weekly Diabetes Log

WEEK OF:		BREAKFAST		LUNCH		DINNER		SNACK #1		SNACK #2		BEDTIME	
		PRE	POST	PRE	POST	PRE	POST	PRE	POST	PRE	POST	PRE	POST
MONDAY	BLOOD SUGAR												
	INSULIN DOSE												
	GRAMS OF CARBS												
	PHYS. ACTIVITY												
TUESDAY	BLOOD SUGAR												
	INSULIN DOSE												
	GRAMS OF CARBS												
	PHYS. ACTIVITY												
WEDNESDAY	BLOOD SUGAR												
	INSULIN DOSE												
	GRAMS OF CARBS												
	PHYS. ACTIVITY												
THURSDAY	BLOOD SUGAR												
	INSULIN DOSE												
	GRAMS OF CARBS												
	PHYS. ACTIVITY												
FRIDAY	BLOOD SUGAR												
	INSULIN DOSE												
	GRAMS OF CARBS												
	PHYS. ACTIVITY												
SATURDAY	BLOOD SUGAR												
	INSULIN DOSE												
	GRAMS OF CARBS												
	PHYS. ACTIVITY												

Weekly Diabetes Log Book

NOTES

MONDAY

TUESDAY

WEDNESDAY

THURSDAY

FRIDAY

SATURDAY

Weekly Diabetes Log

WEEK OF:		BREAKFAST		LUNCH		DINNER		SNACK #1		SNACK #2		BEDTIME	
		PRE	POST	PRE	POST	PRE	POST	PRE	POST	PRE	POST	PRE	POST
MONDAY	BLOOD SUGAR												
	INSULIN DOSE												
	GRAMS OF CARBS												
	PHYS. ACTIVITY												
TUESDAY	BLOOD SUGAR												
	INSULIN DOSE												
	GRAMS OF CARBS												
	PHYS. ACTIVITY												
WEDNESDAY	BLOOD SUGAR												
	INSULIN DOSE												
	GRAMS OF CARBS												
	PHYS. ACTIVITY												
THURSDAY	BLOOD SUGAR												
	INSULIN DOSE												
	GRAMS OF CARBS												
	PHYS. ACTIVITY												
FRIDAY	BLOOD SUGAR												
	INSULIN DOSE												
	GRAMS OF CARBS												
	PHYS. ACTIVITY												
SATURDAY	BLOOD SUGAR												
	INSULIN DOSE												
	GRAMS OF CARBS												
	PHYS. ACTIVITY												

Weekly Diabetes Log Book

NOTES

MONDAY

TUESDAY

WEDNESDAY

THURSDAY

FRIDAY

SATURDAY

Weekly Diabetes Log

WEEK OF:		BREAKFAST		LUNCH		DINNER		SNACK #1		SNACK #2		BEDTIME	
		PRE	POST	PRE	POST	PRE	POST	PRE	POST	PRE	POST	PRE	POST
MONDAY	BLOOD SUGAR												
	INSULIN DOSE												
	GRAMS OF CARBS												
	PHYS. ACTIVITY												
TUESDAY	BLOOD SUGAR												
	INSULIN DOSE												
	GRAMS OF CARBS												
	PHYS. ACTIVITY												
WEDNESDAY	BLOOD SUGAR												
	INSULIN DOSE												
	GRAMS OF CARBS												
	PHYS. ACTIVITY												
THURSDAY	BLOOD SUGAR												
	INSULIN DOSE												
	GRAMS OF CARBS												
	PHYS. ACTIVITY												
FRIDAY	BLOOD SUGAR												
	INSULIN DOSE												
	GRAMS OF CARBS												
	PHYS. ACTIVITY												
SATURDAY	BLOOD SUGAR												
	INSULIN DOSE												
	GRAMS OF CARBS												
	PHYS. ACTIVITY												

Weekly Diabetes Log Book

NOTES

MONDAY

TUESDAY

WEDNESDAY

THURSDAY

FRIDAY

SATURDAY

Weekly Diabetes Log

WEEK OF:		BREAKFAST		LUNCH		DINNER		SNACK #1		SNACK #2		BEDTIME	
		PRE	POST	PRE	POST	PRE	POST	PRE	POST	PRE	POST	PRE	POST
MONDAY	BLOOD SUGAR												
	INSULIN DOSE												
	GRAMS OF CARBS												
	PHYS. ACTIVITY												
TUESDAY	BLOOD SUGAR												
	INSULIN DOSE												
	GRAMS OF CARBS												
	PHYS. ACTIVITY												
WEDNESDAY	BLOOD SUGAR												
	INSULIN DOSE												
	GRAMS OF CARBS												
	PHYS. ACTIVITY												
THURSDAY	BLOOD SUGAR												
	INSULIN DOSE												
	GRAMS OF CARBS												
	PHYS. ACTIVITY												
FRIDAY	BLOOD SUGAR												
	INSULIN DOSE												
	GRAMS OF CARBS												
	PHYS. ACTIVITY												
SATURDAY	BLOOD SUGAR												
	INSULIN DOSE												
	GRAMS OF CARBS												
	PHYS. ACTIVITY												

Weekly Diabetes Log Book

NOTES

MONDAY

TUESDAY

WEDNESDAY

THURSDAY

FRIDAY

SATURDAY

Weekly Diabetes Log

WEEK OF:		BREAKFAST		LUNCH		DINNER		SNACK #1		SNACK #2		BEDTIME	
		PRE	POST	PRE	POST	PRE	POST	PRE	POST	PRE	POST	PRE	POST
MONDAY	BLOOD SUGAR												
	INSULIN DOSE												
	GRAMS OF CARBS												
	PHYS. ACTIVITY												
TUESDAY	BLOOD SUGAR												
	INSULIN DOSE												
	GRAMS OF CARBS												
	PHYS. ACTIVITY												
WEDNESDAY	BLOOD SUGAR												
	INSULIN DOSE												
	GRAMS OF CARBS												
	PHYS. ACTIVITY												
THURSDAY	BLOOD SUGAR												
	INSULIN DOSE												
	GRAMS OF CARBS												
	PHYS. ACTIVITY												
FRIDAY	BLOOD SUGAR												
	INSULIN DOSE												
	GRAMS OF CARBS												
	PHYS. ACTIVITY												
SATURDAY	BLOOD SUGAR												
	INSULIN DOSE												
	GRAMS OF CARBS												
	PHYS. ACTIVITY												

Weekly Diabetes Log Book

NOTES

MONDAY

TUESDAY

WEDNESDAY

THURSDAY

FRIDAY

SATURDAY

Weekly Diabetes Log

WEEK OF:		BREAKFAST		LUNCH		DINNER		SNACK #1		SNACK #2		BEDTIME	
		PRE	POST	PRE	POST	PRE	POST	PRE	POST	PRE	POST	PRE	POST
MONDAY	BLOOD SUGAR												
	INSULIN DOSE												
	GRAMS OF CARBS												
	PHYS. ACTIVITY												
TUESDAY	BLOOD SUGAR												
	INSULIN DOSE												
	GRAMS OF CARBS												
	PHYS. ACTIVITY												
WEDNESDAY	BLOOD SUGAR												
	INSULIN DOSE												
	GRAMS OF CARBS												
	PHYS. ACTIVITY												
THURSDAY	BLOOD SUGAR												
	INSULIN DOSE												
	GRAMS OF CARBS												
	PHYS. ACTIVITY												
FRIDAY	BLOOD SUGAR												
	INSULIN DOSE												
	GRAMS OF CARBS												
	PHYS. ACTIVITY												
SATURDAY	BLOOD SUGAR												
	INSULIN DOSE												
	GRAMS OF CARBS												
	PHYS. ACTIVITY												

Weekly Diabetes Log Book

	NOTES
MONDAY	
TUESDAY	
WEDNESDAY	
THURSDAY	
FRIDAY	
SATURDAY	

Weekly Diabetes Log

WEEK OF:		BREAKFAST		LUNCH		DINNER		SNACK #1		SNACK #2		BEDTIME	
		PRE	POST	PRE	POST	PRE	POST	PRE	POST	PRE	POST	PRE	POST
MONDAY	BLOOD SUGAR												
	INSULIN DOSE												
	GRAMS OF CARBS												
	PHYS. ACTIVITY												
TUESDAY	BLOOD SUGAR												
	INSULIN DOSE												
	GRAMS OF CARBS												
	PHYS. ACTIVITY												
WEDNESDAY	BLOOD SUGAR												
	INSULIN DOSE												
	GRAMS OF CARBS												
	PHYS. ACTIVITY												
THURSDAY	BLOOD SUGAR												
	INSULIN DOSE												
	GRAMS OF CARBS												
	PHYS. ACTIVITY												
FRIDAY	BLOOD SUGAR												
	INSULIN DOSE												
	GRAMS OF CARBS												
	PHYS. ACTIVITY												
SATURDAY	BLOOD SUGAR												
	INSULIN DOSE												
	GRAMS OF CARBS												
	PHYS. ACTIVITY												

Weekly Diabetes Log Book

NOTES

MONDAY

TUESDAY

WEDNESDAY

THURSDAY

FRIDAY

SATURDAY

Weekly Diabetes Log

WEEK OF:		BREAKFAST		LUNCH		DINNER		SNACK #1		SNACK #2		BEDTIME	
		PRE	POST	PRE	POST	PRE	POST	PRE	POST	PRE	POST	PRE	POST
MONDAY	BLOOD SUGAR												
	INSULIN DOSE												
	GRAMS OF CARBS												
	PHYS. ACTIVITY												
TUESDAY	BLOOD SUGAR												
	INSULIN DOSE												
	GRAMS OF CARBS												
	PHYS. ACTIVITY												
WEDNESDAY	BLOOD SUGAR												
	INSULIN DOSE												
	GRAMS OF CARBS												
	PHYS. ACTIVITY												
THURSDAY	BLOOD SUGAR												
	INSULIN DOSE												
	GRAMS OF CARBS												
	PHYS. ACTIVITY												
FRIDAY	BLOOD SUGAR												
	INSULIN DOSE												
	GRAMS OF CARBS												
	PHYS. ACTIVITY												
SATURDAY	BLOOD SUGAR												
	INSULIN DOSE												
	GRAMS OF CARBS												
	PHYS. ACTIVITY												

Weekly Diabetes Log Book

NOTES

MONDAY

TUESDAY

WEDNESDAY

THURSDAY

FRIDAY

SATURDAY

Weekly Diabetes Log

WEEK OF:		BREAKFAST		LUNCH		DINNER		SNACK #1		SNACK #2		BEDTIME	
		PRE	POST	PRE	POST	PRE	POST	PRE	POST	PRE	POST	PRE	POST
MONDAY	BLOOD SUGAR												
	INSULIN DOSE												
	GRAMS OF CARBS												
	PHYS. ACTIVITY												
TUESDAY	BLOOD SUGAR												
	INSULIN DOSE												
	GRAMS OF CARBS												
	PHYS. ACTIVITY												
WEDNESDAY	BLOOD SUGAR												
	INSULIN DOSE												
	GRAMS OF CARBS												
	PHYS. ACTIVITY												
THURSDAY	BLOOD SUGAR												
	INSULIN DOSE												
	GRAMS OF CARBS												
	PHYS. ACTIVITY												
FRIDAY	BLOOD SUGAR												
	INSULIN DOSE												
	GRAMS OF CARBS												
	PHYS. ACTIVITY												
SATURDAY	BLOOD SUGAR												
	INSULIN DOSE												
	GRAMS OF CARBS												
	PHYS. ACTIVITY												

Weekly Diabetes Log Book

NOTES

MONDAY

TUESDAY

WEDNESDAY

THURSDAY

FRIDAY

SATURDAY

Weekly Diabetes Log

WEEK OF:		BREAKFAST		LUNCH		DINNER		SNACK #1		SNACK #2		BEDTIME	
		PRE	POST	PRE	POST	PRE	POST	PRE	POST	PRE	POST	PRE	POST
MONDAY	BLOOD SUGAR												
	INSULIN DOSE												
	GRAMS OF CARBS												
	PHYS. ACTIVITY												
TUESDAY	BLOOD SUGAR												
	INSULIN DOSE												
	GRAMS OF CARBS												
	PHYS. ACTIVITY												
WEDNESDAY	BLOOD SUGAR												
	INSULIN DOSE												
	GRAMS OF CARBS												
	PHYS. ACTIVITY												
THURSDAY	BLOOD SUGAR												
	INSULIN DOSE												
	GRAMS OF CARBS												
	PHYS. ACTIVITY												
FRIDAY	BLOOD SUGAR												
	INSULIN DOSE												
	GRAMS OF CARBS												
	PHYS. ACTIVITY												
SATURDAY	BLOOD SUGAR												
	INSULIN DOSE												
	GRAMS OF CARBS												
	PHYS. ACTIVITY												

Weekly Diabetes Log Book

NOTES

MONDAY

TUESDAY

WEDNESDAY

THURSDAY

FRIDAY

SATURDAY

Weekly Diabetes Log

WEEK OF:		BREAKFAST		LUNCH		DINNER		SNACK #1		SNACK #2		BEDTIME	
		PRE	POST	PRE	POST	PRE	POST	PRE	POST	PRE	POST	PRE	POST
MONDAY	BLOOD SUGAR												
	INSULIN DOSE												
	GRAMS OF CARBS												
	PHYS. ACTIVITY												
TUESDAY	BLOOD SUGAR												
	INSULIN DOSE												
	GRAMS OF CARBS												
	PHYS. ACTIVITY												
WEDNESDAY	BLOOD SUGAR												
	INSULIN DOSE												
	GRAMS OF CARBS												
	PHYS. ACTIVITY												
THURSDAY	BLOOD SUGAR												
	INSULIN DOSE												
	GRAMS OF CARBS												
	PHYS. ACTIVITY												
FRIDAY	BLOOD SUGAR												
	INSULIN DOSE												
	GRAMS OF CARBS												
	PHYS. ACTIVITY												
SATURDAY	BLOOD SUGAR												
	INSULIN DOSE												
	GRAMS OF CARBS												
	PHYS. ACTIVITY												

Weekly Diabetes Log Book

	NOTES
MONDAY	
TUESDAY	
WEDNESDAY	
THURSDAY	
FRIDAY	
SATURDAY	

Weekly Diabetes Log

WEEK OF:		BREAKFAST		LUNCH		DINNER		SNACK #1		SNACK #2		BEDTIME	
		PRE	POST	PRE	POST	PRE	POST	PRE	POST	PRE	POST	PRE	POST
MONDAY	BLOOD SUGAR												
	INSULIN DOSE												
	GRAMS OF CARBS												
	PHYS. ACTIVITY												
TUESDAY	BLOOD SUGAR												
	INSULIN DOSE												
	GRAMS OF CARBS												
	PHYS. ACTIVITY												
WEDNESDAY	BLOOD SUGAR												
	INSULIN DOSE												
	GRAMS OF CARBS												
	PHYS. ACTIVITY												
THURSDAY	BLOOD SUGAR												
	INSULIN DOSE												
	GRAMS OF CARBS												
	PHYS. ACTIVITY												
FRIDAY	BLOOD SUGAR												
	INSULIN DOSE												
	GRAMS OF CARBS												
	PHYS. ACTIVITY												
SATURDAY	BLOOD SUGAR												
	INSULIN DOSE												
	GRAMS OF CARBS												
	PHYS. ACTIVITY												

Weekly Diabetes Log Book

NOTES

MONDAY

TUESDAY

WEDNESDAY

THURSDAY

FRIDAY

SATURDAY

Weekly Diabetes Log

WEEK OF:		BREAKFAST		LUNCH		DINNER		SNACK #1		SNACK #2		BEDTIME	
		PRE	POST	PRE	POST	PRE	POST	PRE	POST	PRE	POST	PRE	POST
MONDAY	BLOOD SUGAR												
	INSULIN DOSE												
	GRAMS OF CARBS												
	PHYS. ACTIVITY												
TUESDAY	BLOOD SUGAR												
	INSULIN DOSE												
	GRAMS OF CARBS												
	PHYS. ACTIVITY												
WEDNESDAY	BLOOD SUGAR												
	INSULIN DOSE												
	GRAMS OF CARBS												
	PHYS. ACTIVITY												
THURSDAY	BLOOD SUGAR												
	INSULIN DOSE												
	GRAMS OF CARBS												
	PHYS. ACTIVITY												
FRIDAY	BLOOD SUGAR												
	INSULIN DOSE												
	GRAMS OF CARBS												
	PHYS. ACTIVITY												
SATURDAY	BLOOD SUGAR												
	INSULIN DOSE												
	GRAMS OF CARBS												
	PHYS. ACTIVITY												

Weekly Diabetes Log Book

NOTES

MONDAY

TUESDAY

WEDNESDAY

THURSDAY

FRIDAY

SATURDAY

Weekly Diabetes Log

WEEK OF:	BREAKFAST		LUNCH		DINNER		SNACK #1		SNACK #2		BEDTIME	
	PRE	POST	PRE	POST	PRE	POST	PRE	POST	PRE	POST	PRE	POST
MONDAY BLOOD SUGAR												
INSULIN DOSE												
GRAMS OF CARBS												
PHYS. ACTIVITY												
TUESDAY BLOOD SUGAR												
INSULIN DOSE												
GRAMS OF CARBS												
PHYS. ACTIVITY												
WEDNESDAY BLOOD SUGAR												
INSULIN DOSE												
GRAMS OF CARBS												
PHYS. ACTIVITY												
THURSDAY BLOOD SUGAR												
INSULIN DOSE												
GRAMS OF CARBS												
PHYS. ACTIVITY												
FRIDAY BLOOD SUGAR												
INSULIN DOSE												
GRAMS OF CARBS												
PHYS. ACTIVITY												
SATURDAY BLOOD SUGAR												
INSULIN DOSE												
GRAMS OF CARBS												
PHYS. ACTIVITY												

Weekly Diabetes Log Book

NOTES

MONDAY

TUESDAY

WEDNESDAY

THURSDAY

FRIDAY

SATURDAY

Weekly Diabetes Log

WEEK OF:		BREAKFAST		LUNCH		DINNER		SNACK #1		SNACK #2		BEDTIME	
		PRE	POST	PRE	POST	PRE	POST	PRE	POST	PRE	POST	PRE	POST
MONDAY	BLOOD SUGAR												
	INSULIN DOSE												
	GRAMS OF CARBS												
	PHYS. ACTIVITY												
TUESDAY	BLOOD SUGAR												
	INSULIN DOSE												
	GRAMS OF CARBS												
	PHYS. ACTIVITY												
WEDNESDAY	BLOOD SUGAR												
	INSULIN DOSE												
	GRAMS OF CARBS												
	PHYS. ACTIVITY												
THURSDAY	BLOOD SUGAR												
	INSULIN DOSE												
	GRAMS OF CARBS												
	PHYS. ACTIVITY												
FRIDAY	BLOOD SUGAR												
	INSULIN DOSE												
	GRAMS OF CARBS												
	PHYS. ACTIVITY												
SATURDAY	BLOOD SUGAR												
	INSULIN DOSE												
	GRAMS OF CARBS												
	PHYS. ACTIVITY												

Weekly Diabetes Log Book

NOTES

MONDAY

TUESDAY

WEDNESDAY

THURSDAY

FRIDAY

SATURDAY

Weekly Diabetes Log

WEEK OF:		BREAKFAST		LUNCH		DINNER		SNACK #1		SNACK #2		BEDTIME	
		PRE	POST	PRE	POST	PRE	POST	PRE	POST	PRE	POST	PRE	POST
MONDAY	BLOOD SUGAR												
	INSULIN DOSE												
	GRAMS OF CARBS												
	PHYS. ACTIVITY												
TUESDAY	BLOOD SUGAR												
	INSULIN DOSE												
	GRAMS OF CARBS												
	PHYS. ACTIVITY												
WEDNESDAY	BLOOD SUGAR												
	INSULIN DOSE												
	GRAMS OF CARBS												
	PHYS. ACTIVITY												
THURSDAY	BLOOD SUGAR												
	INSULIN DOSE												
	GRAMS OF CARBS												
	PHYS. ACTIVITY												
FRIDAY	BLOOD SUGAR												
	INSULIN DOSE												
	GRAMS OF CARBS												
	PHYS. ACTIVITY												
SATURDAY	BLOOD SUGAR												
	INSULIN DOSE												
	GRAMS OF CARBS												
	PHYS. ACTIVITY												

Weekly Diabetes Log Book

NOTES

MONDAY

TUESDAY

WEDNESDAY

THURSDAY

FRIDAY

SATURDAY

Weekly Diabetes Log

WEEK OF:		BREAKFAST		LUNCH		DINNER		SNACK #1		SNACK #2		BEDTIME	
		PRE	POST	PRE	POST	PRE	POST	PRE	POST	PRE	POST	PRE	POST
MONDAY	BLOOD SUGAR												
	INSULIN DOSE												
	GRAMS OF CARBS												
	PHYS. ACTIVITY												
TUESDAY	BLOOD SUGAR												
	INSULIN DOSE												
	GRAMS OF CARBS												
	PHYS. ACTIVITY												
WEDNESDAY	BLOOD SUGAR												
	INSULIN DOSE												
	GRAMS OF CARBS												
	PHYS. ACTIVITY												
THURSDAY	BLOOD SUGAR												
	INSULIN DOSE												
	GRAMS OF CARBS												
	PHYS. ACTIVITY												
FRIDAY	BLOOD SUGAR												
	INSULIN DOSE												
	GRAMS OF CARBS												
	PHYS. ACTIVITY												
SATURDAY	BLOOD SUGAR												
	INSULIN DOSE												
	GRAMS OF CARBS												
	PHYS. ACTIVITY												

Weekly Diabetes Log Book

NOTES

MONDAY

TUESDAY

WEDNESDAY

THURSDAY

FRIDAY

SATURDAY

Weekly Diabetes Log

WEEK OF:		BREAKFAST		LUNCH		DINNER		SNACK #1		SNACK #2		BEDTIME	
		PRE	POST	PRE	POST	PRE	POST	PRE	POST	PRE	POST	PRE	POST
MONDAY	BLOOD SUGAR												
	INSULIN DOSE												
	GRAMS OF CARBS												
	PHYS. ACTIVITY												
TUESDAY	BLOOD SUGAR												
	INSULIN DOSE												
	GRAMS OF CARBS												
	PHYS. ACTIVITY												
WEDNESDAY	BLOOD SUGAR												
	INSULIN DOSE												
	GRAMS OF CARBS												
	PHYS. ACTIVITY												
THURSDAY	BLOOD SUGAR												
	INSULIN DOSE												
	GRAMS OF CARBS												
	PHYS. ACTIVITY												
FRIDAY	BLOOD SUGAR												
	INSULIN DOSE												
	GRAMS OF CARBS												
	PHYS. ACTIVITY												
SATURDAY	BLOOD SUGAR												
	INSULIN DOSE												
	GRAMS OF CARBS												
	PHYS. ACTIVITY												

Weekly Diabetes Log Book

	NOTES
MONDAY	
TUESDAY	
WEDNESDAY	
THURSDAY	
FRIDAY	
SATURDAY	

Weekly Diabetes Log

WEEK OF:		BREAKFAST		LUNCH		DINNER		SNACK #1		SNACK #2		BEDTIME	
		PRE	POST	PRE	POST	PRE	POST	PRE	POST	PRE	POST	PRE	POST
MONDAY	BLOOD SUGAR												
	INSULIN DOSE												
	GRAMS OF CARBS												
	PHYS. ACTIVITY												
TUESDAY	BLOOD SUGAR												
	INSULIN DOSE												
	GRAMS OF CARBS												
	PHYS. ACTIVITY												
WEDNESDAY	BLOOD SUGAR												
	INSULIN DOSE												
	GRAMS OF CARBS												
	PHYS. ACTIVITY												
THURSDAY	BLOOD SUGAR												
	INSULIN DOSE												
	GRAMS OF CARBS												
	PHYS. ACTIVITY												
FRIDAY	BLOOD SUGAR												
	INSULIN DOSE												
	GRAMS OF CARBS												
	PHYS. ACTIVITY												
SATURDAY	BLOOD SUGAR												
	INSULIN DOSE												
	GRAMS OF CARBS												
	PHYS. ACTIVITY												

Weekly Diabetes Log Book

NOTES

MONDAY

TUESDAY

WEDNESDAY

THURSDAY

FRIDAY

SATURDAY

Weekly Diabetes Log

WEEK OF:		BREAKFAST		LUNCH		DINNER		SNACK #1		SNACK #2		BEDTIME	
		PRE	POST	PRE	POST	PRE	POST	PRE	POST	PRE	POST	PRE	POST
MONDAY	BLOOD SUGAR												
	INSULIN DOSE												
	GRAMS OF CARBS												
	PHYS. ACTIVITY												
TUESDAY	BLOOD SUGAR												
	INSULIN DOSE												
	GRAMS OF CARBS												
	PHYS. ACTIVITY												
WEDNESDAY	BLOOD SUGAR												
	INSULIN DOSE												
	GRAMS OF CARBS												
	PHYS. ACTIVITY												
THURSDAY	BLOOD SUGAR												
	INSULIN DOSE												
	GRAMS OF CARBS												
	PHYS. ACTIVITY												
FRIDAY	BLOOD SUGAR												
	INSULIN DOSE												
	GRAMS OF CARBS												
	PHYS. ACTIVITY												
SATURDAY	BLOOD SUGAR												
	INSULIN DOSE												
	GRAMS OF CARBS												
	PHYS. ACTIVITY												

Weekly Diabetes Log Book

NOTES

MONDAY

TUESDAY

WEDNESDAY

THURSDAY

FRIDAY

SATURDAY

Weekly Diabetes Log

WEEK OF:		BREAKFAST		LUNCH		DINNER		SNACK #1		SNACK #2		BEDTIME	
		PRE	POST	PRE	POST	PRE	POST	PRE	POST	PRE	POST	PRE	POST
MONDAY	BLOOD SUGAR												
	INSULIN DOSE												
	GRAMS OF CARBS												
	PHYS. ACTIVITY												
TUESDAY	BLOOD SUGAR												
	INSULIN DOSE												
	GRAMS OF CARBS												
	PHYS. ACTIVITY												
WEDNESDAY	BLOOD SUGAR												
	INSULIN DOSE												
	GRAMS OF CARBS												
	PHYS. ACTIVITY												
THURSDAY	BLOOD SUGAR												
	INSULIN DOSE												
	GRAMS OF CARBS												
	PHYS. ACTIVITY												
FRIDAY	BLOOD SUGAR												
	INSULIN DOSE												
	GRAMS OF CARBS												
	PHYS. ACTIVITY												
SATURDAY	BLOOD SUGAR												
	INSULIN DOSE												
	GRAMS OF CARBS												
	PHYS. ACTIVITY												

Weekly Diabetes Log Book

NOTES

MONDAY

TUESDAY

WEDNESDAY

THURSDAY

FRIDAY

SATURDAY

Weekly Diabetes Log

WEEK OF:		BREAKFAST		LUNCH		DINNER		SNACK #1		SNACK #2		BEDTIME	
		PRE	POST	PRE	POST	PRE	POST	PRE	POST	PRE	POST	PRE	POST
MONDAY	BLOOD SUGAR												
	INSULIN DOSE												
	GRAMS OF CARBS												
	PHYS. ACTIVITY												
TUESDAY	BLOOD SUGAR												
	INSULIN DOSE												
	GRAMS OF CARBS												
	PHYS. ACTIVITY												
WEDNESDAY	BLOOD SUGAR												
	INSULIN DOSE												
	GRAMS OF CARBS												
	PHYS. ACTIVITY												
THURSDAY	BLOOD SUGAR												
	INSULIN DOSE												
	GRAMS OF CARBS												
	PHYS. ACTIVITY												
FRIDAY	BLOOD SUGAR												
	INSULIN DOSE												
	GRAMS OF CARBS												
	PHYS. ACTIVITY												
SATURDAY	BLOOD SUGAR												
	INSULIN DOSE												
	GRAMS OF CARBS												
	PHYS. ACTIVITY												

Weekly Diabetes Log Book

NOTES

MONDAY

TUESDAY

WEDNESDAY

THURSDAY

FRIDAY

SATURDAY

Weekly Diabetes Log

WEEK OF:		BREAKFAST		LUNCH		DINNER		SNACK #1		SNACK #2		BEDTIME	
		PRE	POST	PRE	POST	PRE	POST	PRE	POST	PRE	POST	PRE	POST
MONDAY	BLOOD SUGAR												
	INSULIN DOSE												
	GRAMS OF CARBS												
	PHYS. ACTIVITY												
TUESDAY	BLOOD SUGAR												
	INSULIN DOSE												
	GRAMS OF CARBS												
	PHYS. ACTIVITY												
WEDNESDAY	BLOOD SUGAR												
	INSULIN DOSE												
	GRAMS OF CARBS												
	PHYS. ACTIVITY												
THURSDAY	BLOOD SUGAR												
	INSULIN DOSE												
	GRAMS OF CARBS												
	PHYS. ACTIVITY												
FRIDAY	BLOOD SUGAR												
	INSULIN DOSE												
	GRAMS OF CARBS												
	PHYS. ACTIVITY												
SATURDAY	BLOOD SUGAR												
	INSULIN DOSE												
	GRAMS OF CARBS												
	PHYS. ACTIVITY												

Weekly Diabetes Log Book

NOTES

MONDAY

TUESDAY

WEDNESDAY

THURSDAY

FRIDAY

SATURDAY

Weekly Diabetes Log

WEEK OF:		BREAKFAST		LUNCH		DINNER		SNACK #1		SNACK #2		BEDTIME	
		PRE	POST	PRE	POST	PRE	POST	PRE	POST	PRE	POST	PRE	POST
MONDAY	BLOOD SUGAR												
	INSULIN DOSE												
	GRAMS OF CARBS												
	PHYS. ACTIVITY												
TUESDAY	BLOOD SUGAR												
	INSULIN DOSE												
	GRAMS OF CARBS												
	PHYS. ACTIVITY												
WEDNESDAY	BLOOD SUGAR												
	INSULIN DOSE												
	GRAMS OF CARBS												
	PHYS. ACTIVITY												
THURSDAY	BLOOD SUGAR												
	INSULIN DOSE												
	GRAMS OF CARBS												
	PHYS. ACTIVITY												
FRIDAY	BLOOD SUGAR												
	INSULIN DOSE												
	GRAMS OF CARBS												
	PHYS. ACTIVITY												
SATURDAY	BLOOD SUGAR												
	INSULIN DOSE												
	GRAMS OF CARBS												
	PHYS. ACTIVITY												

Weekly Diabetes Log Book

NOTES

MONDAY

TUESDAY

WEDNESDAY

THURSDAY

FRIDAY

SATURDAY

Weekly Diabetes Log

WEEK OF:		BREAKFAST		LUNCH		DINNER		SNACK #1		SNACK #2		BEDTIME	
		PRE	POST	PRE	POST	PRE	POST	PRE	POST	PRE	POST	PRE	POST
MONDAY	BLOOD SUGAR												
	INSULIN DOSE												
	GRAMS OF CARBS												
	PHYS. ACTIVITY												
TUESDAY	BLOOD SUGAR												
	INSULIN DOSE												
	GRAMS OF CARBS												
	PHYS. ACTIVITY												
WEDNESDAY	BLOOD SUGAR												
	INSULIN DOSE												
	GRAMS OF CARBS												
	PHYS. ACTIVITY												
THURSDAY	BLOOD SUGAR												
	INSULIN DOSE												
	GRAMS OF CARBS												
	PHYS. ACTIVITY												
FRIDAY	BLOOD SUGAR												
	INSULIN DOSE												
	GRAMS OF CARBS												
	PHYS. ACTIVITY												
SATURDAY	BLOOD SUGAR												
	INSULIN DOSE												
	GRAMS OF CARBS												
	PHYS. ACTIVITY												

Weekly Diabetes Log Book

NOTES

MONDAY

TUESDAY

WEDNESDAY

THURSDAY

FRIDAY

SATURDAY

Weekly Diabetes Log

WEEK OF:		BREAKFAST		LUNCH		DINNER		SNACK #1		SNACK #2		BEDTIME	
		PRE	POST	PRE	POST	PRE	POST	PRE	POST	PRE	POST	PRE	POST
MONDAY	BLOOD SUGAR												
	INSULIN DOSE												
	GRAMS OF CARBS												
	PHYS. ACTIVITY												
TUESDAY	BLOOD SUGAR												
	INSULIN DOSE												
	GRAMS OF CARBS												
	PHYS. ACTIVITY												
WEDNESDAY	BLOOD SUGAR												
	INSULIN DOSE												
	GRAMS OF CARBS												
	PHYS. ACTIVITY												
THURSDAY	BLOOD SUGAR												
	INSULIN DOSE												
	GRAMS OF CARBS												
	PHYS. ACTIVITY												
FRIDAY	BLOOD SUGAR												
	INSULIN DOSE												
	GRAMS OF CARBS												
	PHYS. ACTIVITY												
SATURDAY	BLOOD SUGAR												
	INSULIN DOSE												
	GRAMS OF CARBS												
	PHYS. ACTIVITY												

Weekly Diabetes Log Book

NOTES

MONDAY

TUESDAY

WEDNESDAY

THURSDAY

FRIDAY

SATURDAY

Weekly Diabetes Log

WEEK OF:		BREAKFAST		LUNCH		DINNER		SNACK #1		SNACK #2		BEDTIME	
		PRE	POST	PRE	POST	PRE	POST	PRE	POST	PRE	POST	PRE	POST
MONDAY	BLOOD SUGAR												
	INSULIN DOSE												
	GRAMS OF CARBS												
	PHYS. ACTIVITY												
TUESDAY	BLOOD SUGAR												
	INSULIN DOSE												
	GRAMS OF CARBS												
	PHYS. ACTIVITY												
WEDNESDAY	BLOOD SUGAR												
	INSULIN DOSE												
	GRAMS OF CARBS												
	PHYS. ACTIVITY												
THURSDAY	BLOOD SUGAR												
	INSULIN DOSE												
	GRAMS OF CARBS												
	PHYS. ACTIVITY												
FRIDAY	BLOOD SUGAR												
	INSULIN DOSE												
	GRAMS OF CARBS												
	PHYS. ACTIVITY												
SATURDAY	BLOOD SUGAR												
	INSULIN DOSE												
	GRAMS OF CARBS												
	PHYS. ACTIVITY												

Weekly Diabetes Log Book

NOTES

MONDAY

TUESDAY

WEDNESDAY

THURSDAY

FRIDAY

SATURDAY

Weekly Diabetes Log

WEEK OF:		BREAKFAST		LUNCH		DINNER		SNACK #1		SNACK #2		BEDTIME	
		PRE	POST	PRE	POST	PRE	POST	PRE	POST	PRE	POST	PRE	POST
MONDAY	BLOOD SUGAR												
	INSULIN DOSE												
	GRAMS OF CARBS												
	PHYS. ACTIVITY												
TUESDAY	BLOOD SUGAR												
	INSULIN DOSE												
	GRAMS OF CARBS												
	PHYS. ACTIVITY												
WEDNESDAY	BLOOD SUGAR												
	INSULIN DOSE												
	GRAMS OF CARBS												
	PHYS. ACTIVITY												
THURSDAY	BLOOD SUGAR												
	INSULIN DOSE												
	GRAMS OF CARBS												
	PHYS. ACTIVITY												
FRIDAY	BLOOD SUGAR												
	INSULIN DOSE												
	GRAMS OF CARBS												
	PHYS. ACTIVITY												
SATURDAY	BLOOD SUGAR												
	INSULIN DOSE												
	GRAMS OF CARBS												
	PHYS. ACTIVITY												

Weekly Diabetes Log Book

NOTES

MONDAY

TUESDAY

WEDNESDAY

THURSDAY

FRIDAY

SATURDAY

Weekly Diabetes Log

WEEK OF:		BREAKFAST		LUNCH		DINNER		SNACK #1		SNACK #2		BEDTIME	
		PRE	POST	PRE	POST	PRE	POST	PRE	POST	PRE	POST	PRE	POST
MONDAY	BLOOD SUGAR												
	INSULIN DOSE												
	GRAMS OF CARBS												
	PHYS. ACTIVITY												
TUESDAY	BLOOD SUGAR												
	INSULIN DOSE												
	GRAMS OF CARBS												
	PHYS. ACTIVITY												
WEDNESDAY	BLOOD SUGAR												
	INSULIN DOSE												
	GRAMS OF CARBS												
	PHYS. ACTIVITY												
THURSDAY	BLOOD SUGAR												
	INSULIN DOSE												
	GRAMS OF CARBS												
	PHYS. ACTIVITY												
FRIDAY	BLOOD SUGAR												
	INSULIN DOSE												
	GRAMS OF CARBS												
	PHYS. ACTIVITY												
SATURDAY	BLOOD SUGAR												
	INSULIN DOSE												
	GRAMS OF CARBS												
	PHYS. ACTIVITY												

Weekly Diabetes Log Book

NOTES

MONDAY

TUESDAY

WEDNESDAY

THURSDAY

FRIDAY

SATURDAY

Weekly Diabetes Log

WEEK OF:	BREAKFAST		LUNCH		DINNER		SNACK #1		SNACK #2		BEDTIME	
	PRE	POST	PRE	POST	PRE	POST	PRE	POST	PRE	POST	PRE	POST
MONDAY												
BLOOD SUGAR												
INSULIN DOSE												
GRAMS OF CARBS												
PHYS. ACTIVITY												
TUESDAY												
BLOOD SUGAR												
INSULIN DOSE												
GRAMS OF CARBS												
PHYS. ACTIVITY												
WEDNESDAY												
BLOOD SUGAR												
INSULIN DOSE												
GRAMS OF CARBS												
PHYS. ACTIVITY												
THURSDAY												
BLOOD SUGAR												
INSULIN DOSE												
GRAMS OF CARBS												
PHYS. ACTIVITY												
FRIDAY												
BLOOD SUGAR												
INSULIN DOSE												
GRAMS OF CARBS												
PHYS. ACTIVITY												
SATURDAY												
BLOOD SUGAR												
INSULIN DOSE												
GRAMS OF CARBS												
PHYS. ACTIVITY												

Weekly Diabetes Log Book

NOTES

MONDAY

TUESDAY

WEDNESDAY

THURSDAY

FRIDAY

SATURDAY

Weekly Diabetes Log

WEEK OF:		BREAKFAST		LUNCH		DINNER		SNACK #1		SNACK #2		BEDTIME	
		PRE	POST	PRE	POST	PRE	POST	PRE	POST	PRE	POST	PRE	POST
MONDAY	BLOOD SUGAR												
	INSULIN DOSE												
	GRAMS OF CARBS												
	PHYS. ACTIVITY												
TUESDAY	BLOOD SUGAR												
	INSULIN DOSE												
	GRAMS OF CARBS												
	PHYS. ACTIVITY												
WEDNESDAY	BLOOD SUGAR												
	INSULIN DOSE												
	GRAMS OF CARBS												
	PHYS. ACTIVITY												
THURSDAY	BLOOD SUGAR												
	INSULIN DOSE												
	GRAMS OF CARBS												
	PHYS. ACTIVITY												
FRIDAY	BLOOD SUGAR												
	INSULIN DOSE												
	GRAMS OF CARBS												
	PHYS. ACTIVITY												
SATURDAY	BLOOD SUGAR												
	INSULIN DOSE												
	GRAMS OF CARBS												
	PHYS. ACTIVITY												

Weekly Diabetes Log Book

NOTES

MONDAY

TUESDAY

WEDNESDAY

THURSDAY

FRIDAY

SATURDAY

Weekly Diabetes Log

WEEK OF:		BREAKFAST		LUNCH		DINNER		SNACK #1		SNACK #2		BEDTIME	
		PRE	POST	PRE	POST	PRE	POST	PRE	POST	PRE	POST	PRE	POST
MONDAY	BLOOD SUGAR												
	INSULIN DOSE												
	GRAMS OF CARBS												
	PHYS. ACTIVITY												
TUESDAY	BLOOD SUGAR												
	INSULIN DOSE												
	GRAMS OF CARBS												
	PHYS. ACTIVITY												
WEDNESDAY	BLOOD SUGAR												
	INSULIN DOSE												
	GRAMS OF CARBS												
	PHYS. ACTIVITY												
THURSDAY	BLOOD SUGAR												
	INSULIN DOSE												
	GRAMS OF CARBS												
	PHYS. ACTIVITY												
FRIDAY	BLOOD SUGAR												
	INSULIN DOSE												
	GRAMS OF CARBS												
	PHYS. ACTIVITY												
SATURDAY	BLOOD SUGAR												
	INSULIN DOSE												
	GRAMS OF CARBS												
	PHYS. ACTIVITY												

Weekly Diabetes Log Book

NOTES

MONDAY

TUESDAY

WEDNESDAY

THURSDAY

FRIDAY

SATURDAY

Weekly Diabetes Log

WEEK OF:		BREAKFAST		LUNCH		DINNER		SNACK #1		SNACK #2		BEDTIME	
		PRE	POST	PRE	POST	PRE	POST	PRE	POST	PRE	POST	PRE	POST
MONDAY	BLOOD SUGAR												
	INSULIN DOSE												
	GRAMS OF CARBS												
	PHYS. ACTIVITY												
TUESDAY	BLOOD SUGAR												
	INSULIN DOSE												
	GRAMS OF CARBS												
	PHYS. ACTIVITY												
WEDNESDAY	BLOOD SUGAR												
	INSULIN DOSE												
	GRAMS OF CARBS												
	PHYS. ACTIVITY												
THURSDAY	BLOOD SUGAR												
	INSULIN DOSE												
	GRAMS OF CARBS												
	PHYS. ACTIVITY												
FRIDAY	BLOOD SUGAR												
	INSULIN DOSE												
	GRAMS OF CARBS												
	PHYS. ACTIVITY												
SATURDAY	BLOOD SUGAR												
	INSULIN DOSE												
	GRAMS OF CARBS												
	PHYS. ACTIVITY												

Weekly Diabetes Log Book

NOTES

MONDAY

TUESDAY

WEDNESDAY

THURSDAY

FRIDAY

SATURDAY

Weekly Diabetes Log

WEEK OF:		BREAKFAST		LUNCH		DINNER		SNACK #1		SNACK #2		BEDTIME	
		PRE	POST	PRE	POST	PRE	POST	PRE	POST	PRE	POST	PRE	POST
MONDAY	BLOOD SUGAR												
	INSULIN DOSE												
	GRAMS OF CARBS												
	PHYS. ACTIVITY												
TUESDAY	BLOOD SUGAR												
	INSULIN DOSE												
	GRAMS OF CARBS												
	PHYS. ACTIVITY												
WEDNESDAY	BLOOD SUGAR												
	INSULIN DOSE												
	GRAMS OF CARBS												
	PHYS. ACTIVITY												
THURSDAY	BLOOD SUGAR												
	INSULIN DOSE												
	GRAMS OF CARBS												
	PHYS. ACTIVITY												
FRIDAY	BLOOD SUGAR												
	INSULIN DOSE												
	GRAMS OF CARBS												
	PHYS. ACTIVITY												
SATURDAY	BLOOD SUGAR												
	INSULIN DOSE												
	GRAMS OF CARBS												
	PHYS. ACTIVITY												

Weekly Diabetes Log Book

NOTES

MONDAY

TUESDAY

WEDNESDAY

THURSDAY

FRIDAY

SATURDAY

Weekly Diabetes Log

WEEK OF:	BREAKFAST		LUNCH		DINNER		SNACK #1		SNACK #2		BEDTIME	
	PRE	POST	PRE	POST	PRE	POST	PRE	POST	PRE	POST	PRE	POST

MONDAY
BLOOD SUGAR												
INSULIN DOSE												
GRAMS OF CARBS												
PHYS. ACTIVITY												

TUESDAY
BLOOD SUGAR												
INSULIN DOSE												
GRAMS OF CARBS												
PHYS. ACTIVITY												

WEDNESDAY
BLOOD SUGAR												
INSULIN DOSE												
GRAMS OF CARBS												
PHYS. ACTIVITY												

THURSDAY
BLOOD SUGAR												
INSULIN DOSE												
GRAMS OF CARBS												
PHYS. ACTIVITY												

FRIDAY
BLOOD SUGAR												
INSULIN DOSE												
GRAMS OF CARBS												
PHYS. ACTIVITY												

SATURDAY
BLOOD SUGAR												
INSULIN DOSE												
GRAMS OF CARBS												
PHYS. ACTIVITY												

Weekly Diabetes Log Book

NOTES

MONDAY

TUESDAY

WEDNESDAY

THURSDAY

FRIDAY

SATURDAY

Weekly Diabetes Log

WEEK OF:		BREAKFAST		LUNCH		DINNER		SNACK #1		SNACK #2		BEDTIME	
		PRE	POST	PRE	POST	PRE	POST	PRE	POST	PRE	POST	PRE	POST
MONDAY	BLOOD SUGAR												
	INSULIN DOSE												
	GRAMS OF CARBS												
	PHYS. ACTIVITY												
TUESDAY	BLOOD SUGAR												
	INSULIN DOSE												
	GRAMS OF CARBS												
	PHYS. ACTIVITY												
WEDNESDAY	BLOOD SUGAR												
	INSULIN DOSE												
	GRAMS OF CARBS												
	PHYS. ACTIVITY												
THURSDAY	BLOOD SUGAR												
	INSULIN DOSE												
	GRAMS OF CARBS												
	PHYS. ACTIVITY												
FRIDAY	BLOOD SUGAR												
	INSULIN DOSE												
	GRAMS OF CARBS												
	PHYS. ACTIVITY												
SATURDAY	BLOOD SUGAR												
	INSULIN DOSE												
	GRAMS OF CARBS												
	PHYS. ACTIVITY												

Weekly Diabetes Log Book

	NOTES
MONDAY	
TUESDAY	
WEDNESDAY	
THURSDAY	
FRIDAY	
SATURDAY	

Weekly Diabetes Log

WEEK OF:		BREAKFAST		LUNCH		DINNER		SNACK #1		SNACK #2		BEDTIME	
		PRE	POST	PRE	POST	PRE	POST	PRE	POST	PRE	POST	PRE	POST
MONDAY	BLOOD SUGAR												
	INSULIN DOSE												
	GRAMS OF CARBS												
	PHYS. ACTIVITY												
TUESDAY	BLOOD SUGAR												
	INSULIN DOSE												
	GRAMS OF CARBS												
	PHYS. ACTIVITY												
WEDNESDAY	BLOOD SUGAR												
	INSULIN DOSE												
	GRAMS OF CARBS												
	PHYS. ACTIVITY												
THURSDAY	BLOOD SUGAR												
	INSULIN DOSE												
	GRAMS OF CARBS												
	PHYS. ACTIVITY												
FRIDAY	BLOOD SUGAR												
	INSULIN DOSE												
	GRAMS OF CARBS												
	PHYS. ACTIVITY												
SATURDAY	BLOOD SUGAR												
	INSULIN DOSE												
	GRAMS OF CARBS												
	PHYS. ACTIVITY												

Weekly Diabetes Log Book

NOTES

MONDAY

TUESDAY

WEDNESDAY

THURSDAY

FRIDAY

SATURDAY

Weekly Diabetes Log

WEEK OF:		BREAKFAST		LUNCH		DINNER		SNACK #1		SNACK #2		BEDTIME	
		PRE	POST	PRE	POST	PRE	POST	PRE	POST	PRE	POST	PRE	POST
MONDAY	BLOOD SUGAR												
	INSULIN DOSE												
	GRAMS OF CARBS												
	PHYS. ACTIVITY												
TUESDAY	BLOOD SUGAR												
	INSULIN DOSE												
	GRAMS OF CARBS												
	PHYS. ACTIVITY												
WEDNESDAY	BLOOD SUGAR												
	INSULIN DOSE												
	GRAMS OF CARBS												
	PHYS. ACTIVITY												
THURSDAY	BLOOD SUGAR												
	INSULIN DOSE												
	GRAMS OF CARBS												
	PHYS. ACTIVITY												
FRIDAY	BLOOD SUGAR												
	INSULIN DOSE												
	GRAMS OF CARBS												
	PHYS. ACTIVITY												
SATURDAY	BLOOD SUGAR												
	INSULIN DOSE												
	GRAMS OF CARBS												
	PHYS. ACTIVITY												

Weekly Diabetes Log Book

	NOTES
MONDAY	
TUESDAY	
WEDNESDAY	
THURSDAY	
FRIDAY	
SATURDAY	

Weekly Diabetes Log

WEEK OF:		BREAKFAST		LUNCH		DINNER		SNACK #1		SNACK #2		BEDTIME	
		PRE	POST	PRE	POST	PRE	POST	PRE	POST	PRE	POST	PRE	POST
MONDAY	BLOOD SUGAR												
	INSULIN DOSE												
	GRAMS OF CARBS												
	PHYS. ACTIVITY												
TUESDAY	BLOOD SUGAR												
	INSULIN DOSE												
	GRAMS OF CARBS												
	PHYS. ACTIVITY												
WEDNESDAY	BLOOD SUGAR												
	INSULIN DOSE												
	GRAMS OF CARBS												
	PHYS. ACTIVITY												
THURSDAY	BLOOD SUGAR												
	INSULIN DOSE												
	GRAMS OF CARBS												
	PHYS. ACTIVITY												
FRIDAY	BLOOD SUGAR												
	INSULIN DOSE												
	GRAMS OF CARBS												
	PHYS. ACTIVITY												
SATURDAY	BLOOD SUGAR												
	INSULIN DOSE												
	GRAMS OF CARBS												
	PHYS. ACTIVITY												

Weekly Diabetes Log Book

NOTES

MONDAY

TUESDAY

WEDNESDAY

THURSDAY

FRIDAY

SATURDAY

Weekly Diabetes Log

WEEK OF:		BREAKFAST		LUNCH		DINNER		SNACK #1		SNACK #2		BEDTIME	
		PRE	POST	PRE	POST	PRE	POST	PRE	POST	PRE	POST	PRE	POST
MONDAY	BLOOD SUGAR												
	INSULIN DOSE												
	GRAMS OF CARBS												
	PHYS. ACTIVITY												
TUESDAY	BLOOD SUGAR												
	INSULIN DOSE												
	GRAMS OF CARBS												
	PHYS. ACTIVITY												
WEDNESDAY	BLOOD SUGAR												
	INSULIN DOSE												
	GRAMS OF CARBS												
	PHYS. ACTIVITY												
THURSDAY	BLOOD SUGAR												
	INSULIN DOSE												
	GRAMS OF CARBS												
	PHYS. ACTIVITY												
FRIDAY	BLOOD SUGAR												
	INSULIN DOSE												
	GRAMS OF CARBS												
	PHYS. ACTIVITY												
SATURDAY	BLOOD SUGAR												
	INSULIN DOSE												
	GRAMS OF CARBS												
	PHYS. ACTIVITY												

Weekly Diabetes Log Book

NOTES

MONDAY

TUESDAY

WEDNESDAY

THURSDAY

FRIDAY

SATURDAY

Weekly Diabetes Log

WEEK OF:		BREAKFAST		LUNCH		DINNER		SNACK #1		SNACK #2		BEDTIME	
		PRE	POST	PRE	POST	PRE	POST	PRE	POST	PRE	POST	PRE	POST
MONDAY	BLOOD SUGAR												
	INSULIN DOSE												
	GRAMS OF CARBS												
	PHYS. ACTIVITY												
TUESDAY	BLOOD SUGAR												
	INSULIN DOSE												
	GRAMS OF CARBS												
	PHYS. ACTIVITY												
WEDNESDAY	BLOOD SUGAR												
	INSULIN DOSE												
	GRAMS OF CARBS												
	PHYS. ACTIVITY												
THURSDAY	BLOOD SUGAR												
	INSULIN DOSE												
	GRAMS OF CARBS												
	PHYS. ACTIVITY												
FRIDAY	BLOOD SUGAR												
	INSULIN DOSE												
	GRAMS OF CARBS												
	PHYS. ACTIVITY												
SATURDAY	BLOOD SUGAR												
	INSULIN DOSE												
	GRAMS OF CARBS												
	PHYS. ACTIVITY												

Weekly Diabetes Log Book

NOTES

MONDAY

TUESDAY

WEDNESDAY

THURSDAY

FRIDAY

SATURDAY

Weekly Diabetes Log

WEEK OF:		BREAKFAST		LUNCH		DINNER		SNACK #1		SNACK #2		BEDTIME	
		PRE	POST	PRE	POST	PRE	POST	PRE	POST	PRE	POST	PRE	POST
MONDAY	BLOOD SUGAR												
	INSULIN DOSE												
	GRAMS OF CARBS												
	PHYS. ACTIVITY												
TUESDAY	BLOOD SUGAR												
	INSULIN DOSE												
	GRAMS OF CARBS												
	PHYS. ACTIVITY												
WEDNESDAY	BLOOD SUGAR												
	INSULIN DOSE												
	GRAMS OF CARBS												
	PHYS. ACTIVITY												
THURSDAY	BLOOD SUGAR												
	INSULIN DOSE												
	GRAMS OF CARBS												
	PHYS. ACTIVITY												
FRIDAY	BLOOD SUGAR												
	INSULIN DOSE												
	GRAMS OF CARBS												
	PHYS. ACTIVITY												
SATURDAY	BLOOD SUGAR												
	INSULIN DOSE												
	GRAMS OF CARBS												
	PHYS. ACTIVITY												

Weekly Diabetes Log Book

NOTES

MONDAY

TUESDAY

WEDNESDAY

THURSDAY

FRIDAY

SATURDAY

Weekly Diabetes Log

WEEK OF:		BREAKFAST		LUNCH		DINNER		SNACK #1		SNACK #2		BEDTIME	
		PRE	POST	PRE	POST	PRE	POST	PRE	POST	PRE	POST	PRE	POST
MONDAY	BLOOD SUGAR												
	INSULIN DOSE												
	GRAMS OF CARBS												
	PHYS. ACTIVITY												
TUESDAY	BLOOD SUGAR												
	INSULIN DOSE												
	GRAMS OF CARBS												
	PHYS. ACTIVITY												
WEDNESDAY	BLOOD SUGAR												
	INSULIN DOSE												
	GRAMS OF CARBS												
	PHYS. ACTIVITY												
THURSDAY	BLOOD SUGAR												
	INSULIN DOSE												
	GRAMS OF CARBS												
	PHYS. ACTIVITY												
FRIDAY	BLOOD SUGAR												
	INSULIN DOSE												
	GRAMS OF CARBS												
	PHYS. ACTIVITY												
SATURDAY	BLOOD SUGAR												
	INSULIN DOSE												
	GRAMS OF CARBS												
	PHYS. ACTIVITY												

Weekly Diabetes Log Book

NOTES

MONDAY

TUESDAY

WEDNESDAY

THURSDAY

FRIDAY

SATURDAY

Weekly Diabetes Log

WEEK OF:	BREAKFAST		LUNCH		DINNER		SNACK #1		SNACK #2		BEDTIME	
	PRE	POST	PRE	POST	PRE	POST	PRE	POST	PRE	POST	PRE	POST

MONDAY

	BREAKFAST		LUNCH		DINNER		SNACK #1		SNACK #2		BEDTIME	
BLOOD SUGAR												
INSULIN DOSE												
GRAMS OF CARBS												
PHYS. ACTIVITY												

TUESDAY

	BREAKFAST		LUNCH		DINNER		SNACK #1		SNACK #2		BEDTIME	
BLOOD SUGAR												
INSULIN DOSE												
GRAMS OF CARBS												
PHYS. ACTIVITY												

WEDNESDAY

	BREAKFAST		LUNCH		DINNER		SNACK #1		SNACK #2		BEDTIME	
BLOOD SUGAR												
INSULIN DOSE												
GRAMS OF CARBS												
PHYS. ACTIVITY												

THURSDAY

	BREAKFAST		LUNCH		DINNER		SNACK #1		SNACK #2		BEDTIME	
BLOOD SUGAR												
INSULIN DOSE												
GRAMS OF CARBS												
PHYS. ACTIVITY												

FRIDAY

	BREAKFAST		LUNCH		DINNER		SNACK #1		SNACK #2		BEDTIME	
BLOOD SUGAR												
INSULIN DOSE												
GRAMS OF CARBS												
PHYS. ACTIVITY												

SATURDAY

	BREAKFAST		LUNCH		DINNER		SNACK #1		SNACK #2		BEDTIME	
BLOOD SUGAR												
INSULIN DOSE												
GRAMS OF CARBS												
PHYS. ACTIVITY												

Weekly Diabetes Log Book

NOTES

MONDAY

TUESDAY

WEDNESDAY

THURSDAY

FRIDAY

SATURDAY

Weekly Diabetes Log

WEEK OF:	BREAKFAST		LUNCH		DINNER		SNACK #1		SNACK #2		BEDTIME	
	PRE	POST	PRE	POST	PRE	POST	PRE	POST	PRE	POST	PRE	POST
MONDAY BLOOD SUGAR												
INSULIN DOSE												
GRAMS OF CARBS												
PHYS. ACTIVITY												
TUESDAY BLOOD SUGAR												
INSULIN DOSE												
GRAMS OF CARBS												
PHYS. ACTIVITY												
WEDNESDAY BLOOD SUGAR												
INSULIN DOSE												
GRAMS OF CARBS												
PHYS. ACTIVITY												
THURSDAY BLOOD SUGAR												
INSULIN DOSE												
GRAMS OF CARBS												
PHYS. ACTIVITY												
FRIDAY BLOOD SUGAR												
INSULIN DOSE												
GRAMS OF CARBS												
PHYS. ACTIVITY												
SATURDAY BLOOD SUGAR												
INSULIN DOSE												
GRAMS OF CARBS												
PHYS. ACTIVITY												

Weekly Diabetes Log Book

NOTES

MONDAY

TUESDAY

WEDNESDAY

THURSDAY

FRIDAY

SATURDAY

Weekly Diabetes Log

WEEK OF:		BREAKFAST		LUNCH		DINNER		SNACK #1		SNACK #2		BEDTIME	
		PRE	POST	PRE	POST	PRE	POST	PRE	POST	PRE	POST	PRE	POST
MONDAY	BLOOD SUGAR												
	INSULIN DOSE												
	GRAMS OF CARBS												
	PHYS. ACTIVITY												
TUESDAY	BLOOD SUGAR												
	INSULIN DOSE												
	GRAMS OF CARBS												
	PHYS. ACTIVITY												
WEDNESDAY	BLOOD SUGAR												
	INSULIN DOSE												
	GRAMS OF CARBS												
	PHYS. ACTIVITY												
THURSDAY	BLOOD SUGAR												
	INSULIN DOSE												
	GRAMS OF CARBS												
	PHYS. ACTIVITY												
FRIDAY	BLOOD SUGAR												
	INSULIN DOSE												
	GRAMS OF CARBS												
	PHYS. ACTIVITY												
SATURDAY	BLOOD SUGAR												
	INSULIN DOSE												
	GRAMS OF CARBS												
	PHYS. ACTIVITY												

Weekly Diabetes Log Book

NOTES

MONDAY

TUESDAY

WEDNESDAY

THURSDAY

FRIDAY

SATURDAY

Weekly Diabetes Log

WEEK OF:		BREAKFAST		LUNCH		DINNER		SNACK #1		SNACK #2		BEDTIME	
		PRE	POST	PRE	POST	PRE	POST	PRE	POST	PRE	POST	PRE	POST
MONDAY	BLOOD SUGAR												
	INSULIN DOSE												
	GRAMS OF CARBS												
	PHYS. ACTIVITY												
TUESDAY	BLOOD SUGAR												
	INSULIN DOSE												
	GRAMS OF CARBS												
	PHYS. ACTIVITY												
WEDNESDAY	BLOOD SUGAR												
	INSULIN DOSE												
	GRAMS OF CARBS												
	PHYS. ACTIVITY												
THURSDAY	BLOOD SUGAR												
	INSULIN DOSE												
	GRAMS OF CARBS												
	PHYS. ACTIVITY												
FRIDAY	BLOOD SUGAR												
	INSULIN DOSE												
	GRAMS OF CARBS												
	PHYS. ACTIVITY												
SATURDAY	BLOOD SUGAR												
	INSULIN DOSE												
	GRAMS OF CARBS												
	PHYS. ACTIVITY												

Weekly Diabetes Log Book

NOTES

MONDAY

TUESDAY

WEDNESDAY

THURSDAY

FRIDAY

SATURDAY

Weekly Diabetes Log

WEEK OF:		BREAKFAST		LUNCH		DINNER		SNACK #1		SNACK #2		BEDTIME	
		PRE	POST	PRE	POST	PRE	POST	PRE	POST	PRE	POST	PRE	POST
MONDAY	BLOOD SUGAR												
	INSULIN DOSE												
	GRAMS OF CARBS												
	PHYS. ACTIVITY												
TUESDAY	BLOOD SUGAR												
	INSULIN DOSE												
	GRAMS OF CARBS												
	PHYS. ACTIVITY												
WEDNESDAY	BLOOD SUGAR												
	INSULIN DOSE												
	GRAMS OF CARBS												
	PHYS. ACTIVITY												
THURSDAY	BLOOD SUGAR												
	INSULIN DOSE												
	GRAMS OF CARBS												
	PHYS. ACTIVITY												
FRIDAY	BLOOD SUGAR												
	INSULIN DOSE												
	GRAMS OF CARBS												
	PHYS. ACTIVITY												
SATURDAY	BLOOD SUGAR												
	INSULIN DOSE												
	GRAMS OF CARBS												
	PHYS. ACTIVITY												

Weekly Diabetes Log Book

NOTES

MONDAY

TUESDAY

WEDNESDAY

THURSDAY

FRIDAY

SATURDAY

Weekly Diabetes Log

WEEK OF:		BREAKFAST		LUNCH		DINNER		SNACK #1		SNACK #2		BEDTIME	
		PRE	POST	PRE	POST	PRE	POST	PRE	POST	PRE	POST	PRE	POST
MONDAY	BLOOD SUGAR												
	INSULIN DOSE												
	GRAMS OF CARBS												
	PHYS. ACTIVITY												
TUESDAY	BLOOD SUGAR												
	INSULIN DOSE												
	GRAMS OF CARBS												
	PHYS. ACTIVITY												
WEDNESDAY	BLOOD SUGAR												
	INSULIN DOSE												
	GRAMS OF CARBS												
	PHYS. ACTIVITY												
THURSDAY	BLOOD SUGAR												
	INSULIN DOSE												
	GRAMS OF CARBS												
	PHYS. ACTIVITY												
FRIDAY	BLOOD SUGAR												
	INSULIN DOSE												
	GRAMS OF CARBS												
	PHYS. ACTIVITY												
SATURDAY	BLOOD SUGAR												
	INSULIN DOSE												
	GRAMS OF CARBS												
	PHYS. ACTIVITY												

Weekly Diabetes Log Book

NOTES

MONDAY

TUESDAY

WEDNESDAY

THURSDAY

FRIDAY

SATURDAY

Weekly Diabetes Log

WEEK OF:		BREAKFAST		LUNCH		DINNER		SNACK #1		SNACK #2		BEDTIME	
		PRE	POST	PRE	POST	PRE	POST	PRE	POST	PRE	POST	PRE	POST
MONDAY	BLOOD SUGAR												
	INSULIN DOSE												
	GRAMS OF CARBS												
	PHYS. ACTIVITY												
TUESDAY	BLOOD SUGAR												
	INSULIN DOSE												
	GRAMS OF CARBS												
	PHYS. ACTIVITY												
WEDNESDAY	BLOOD SUGAR												
	INSULIN DOSE												
	GRAMS OF CARBS												
	PHYS. ACTIVITY												
THURSDAY	BLOOD SUGAR												
	INSULIN DOSE												
	GRAMS OF CARBS												
	PHYS. ACTIVITY												
FRIDAY	BLOOD SUGAR												
	INSULIN DOSE												
	GRAMS OF CARBS												
	PHYS. ACTIVITY												
SATURDAY	BLOOD SUGAR												
	INSULIN DOSE												
	GRAMS OF CARBS												
	PHYS. ACTIVITY												

Weekly Diabetes Log Book

NOTES

MONDAY

TUESDAY

WEDNESDAY

THURSDAY

FRIDAY

SATURDAY

Weekly Diabetes Log

WEEK OF:		BREAKFAST		LUNCH		DINNER		SNACK #1		SNACK #2		BEDTIME	
		PRE	POST	PRE	POST	PRE	POST	PRE	POST	PRE	POST	PRE	POST
MONDAY	BLOOD SUGAR												
	INSULIN DOSE												
	GRAMS OF CARBS												
	PHYS. ACTIVITY												
TUESDAY	BLOOD SUGAR												
	INSULIN DOSE												
	GRAMS OF CARBS												
	PHYS. ACTIVITY												
WEDNESDAY	BLOOD SUGAR												
	INSULIN DOSE												
	GRAMS OF CARBS												
	PHYS. ACTIVITY												
THURSDAY	BLOOD SUGAR												
	INSULIN DOSE												
	GRAMS OF CARBS												
	PHYS. ACTIVITY												
FRIDAY	BLOOD SUGAR												
	INSULIN DOSE												
	GRAMS OF CARBS												
	PHYS. ACTIVITY												
SATURDAY	BLOOD SUGAR												
	INSULIN DOSE												
	GRAMS OF CARBS												
	PHYS. ACTIVITY												

Weekly Diabetes Log Book

NOTES

MONDAY

TUESDAY

WEDNESDAY

THURSDAY

FRIDAY

SATURDAY

Weekly Diabetes Log

WEEK OF:	BREAKFAST		LUNCH		DINNER		SNACK #1		SNACK #2		BEDTIME	
	PRE	POST	PRE	POST	PRE	POST	PRE	POST	PRE	POST	PRE	POST

MONDAY
BLOOD SUGAR												
INSULIN DOSE												
GRAMS OF CARBS												
PHYS. ACTIVITY												

TUESDAY
BLOOD SUGAR												
INSULIN DOSE												
GRAMS OF CARBS												
PHYS. ACTIVITY												

WEDNESDAY
BLOOD SUGAR												
INSULIN DOSE												
GRAMS OF CARBS												
PHYS. ACTIVITY												

THURSDAY
BLOOD SUGAR												
INSULIN DOSE												
GRAMS OF CARBS												
PHYS. ACTIVITY												

FRIDAY
BLOOD SUGAR												
INSULIN DOSE												
GRAMS OF CARBS												
PHYS. ACTIVITY												

SATURDAY
BLOOD SUGAR												
INSULIN DOSE												
GRAMS OF CARBS												
PHYS. ACTIVITY												

Weekly Diabetes Log Book

NOTES

MONDAY

TUESDAY

WEDNESDAY

THURSDAY

FRIDAY

SATURDAY

Weekly Diabetes Log

WEEK OF:		BREAKFAST		LUNCH		DINNER		SNACK #1		SNACK #2		BEDTIME	
		PRE	POST	PRE	POST	PRE	POST	PRE	POST	PRE	POST	PRE	POST
MONDAY	BLOOD SUGAR												
	INSULIN DOSE												
	GRAMS OF CARBS												
	PHYS. ACTIVITY												
TUESDAY	BLOOD SUGAR												
	INSULIN DOSE												
	GRAMS OF CARBS												
	PHYS. ACTIVITY												
WEDNESDAY	BLOOD SUGAR												
	INSULIN DOSE												
	GRAMS OF CARBS												
	PHYS. ACTIVITY												
THURSDAY	BLOOD SUGAR												
	INSULIN DOSE												
	GRAMS OF CARBS												
	PHYS. ACTIVITY												
FRIDAY	BLOOD SUGAR												
	INSULIN DOSE												
	GRAMS OF CARBS												
	PHYS. ACTIVITY												
SATURDAY	BLOOD SUGAR												
	INSULIN DOSE												
	GRAMS OF CARBS												
	PHYS. ACTIVITY												

Weekly Diabetes Log Book

NOTES

MONDAY

TUESDAY

WEDNESDAY

THURSDAY

FRIDAY

SATURDAY

Weekly Diabetes Log

WEEK OF:		BREAKFAST		LUNCH		DINNER		SNACK #1		SNACK #2		BEDTIME	
		PRE	POST	PRE	POST	PRE	POST	PRE	POST	PRE	POST	PRE	POST
MONDAY	BLOOD SUGAR												
	INSULIN DOSE												
	GRAMS OF CARBS												
	PHYS. ACTIVITY												
TUESDAY	BLOOD SUGAR												
	INSULIN DOSE												
	GRAMS OF CARBS												
	PHYS. ACTIVITY												
WEDNESDAY	BLOOD SUGAR												
	INSULIN DOSE												
	GRAMS OF CARBS												
	PHYS. ACTIVITY												
THURSDAY	BLOOD SUGAR												
	INSULIN DOSE												
	GRAMS OF CARBS												
	PHYS. ACTIVITY												
FRIDAY	BLOOD SUGAR												
	INSULIN DOSE												
	GRAMS OF CARBS												
	PHYS. ACTIVITY												
SATURDAY	BLOOD SUGAR												
	INSULIN DOSE												
	GRAMS OF CARBS												
	PHYS. ACTIVITY												

Weekly Diabetes Log Book

NOTES

MONDAY

TUESDAY

WEDNESDAY

THURSDAY

FRIDAY

SATURDAY

Weekly Diabetes Log

WEEK OF:		BREAKFAST		LUNCH		DINNER		SNACK #1		SNACK #2		BEDTIME	
		PRE	POST	PRE	POST	PRE	POST	PRE	POST	PRE	POST	PRE	POST
MONDAY	BLOOD SUGAR												
	INSULIN DOSE												
	GRAMS OF CARBS												
	PHYS. ACTIVITY												
TUESDAY	BLOOD SUGAR												
	INSULIN DOSE												
	GRAMS OF CARBS												
	PHYS. ACTIVITY												
WEDNESDAY	BLOOD SUGAR												
	INSULIN DOSE												
	GRAMS OF CARBS												
	PHYS. ACTIVITY												
THURSDAY	BLOOD SUGAR												
	INSULIN DOSE												
	GRAMS OF CARBS												
	PHYS. ACTIVITY												
FRIDAY	BLOOD SUGAR												
	INSULIN DOSE												
	GRAMS OF CARBS												
	PHYS. ACTIVITY												
SATURDAY	BLOOD SUGAR												
	INSULIN DOSE												
	GRAMS OF CARBS												
	PHYS. ACTIVITY												

Weekly Diabetes Log Book

NOTES

MONDAY

TUESDAY

WEDNESDAY

THURSDAY

FRIDAY

SATURDAY

Weekly Diabetes Log

WEEK OF:		BREAKFAST		LUNCH		DINNER		SNACK #1		SNACK #2		BEDTIME	
		PRE	POST	PRE	POST	PRE	POST	PRE	POST	PRE	POST	PRE	POST
MONDAY	BLOOD SUGAR												
	INSULIN DOSE												
	GRAMS OF CARBS												
	PHYS. ACTIVITY												
TUESDAY	BLOOD SUGAR												
	INSULIN DOSE												
	GRAMS OF CARBS												
	PHYS. ACTIVITY												
WEDNESDAY	BLOOD SUGAR												
	INSULIN DOSE												
	GRAMS OF CARBS												
	PHYS. ACTIVITY												
THURSDAY	BLOOD SUGAR												
	INSULIN DOSE												
	GRAMS OF CARBS												
	PHYS. ACTIVITY												
FRIDAY	BLOOD SUGAR												
	INSULIN DOSE												
	GRAMS OF CARBS												
	PHYS. ACTIVITY												
SATURDAY	BLOOD SUGAR												
	INSULIN DOSE												
	GRAMS OF CARBS												
	PHYS. ACTIVITY												

Weekly Diabetes Log Book

NOTES

MONDAY

TUESDAY

WEDNESDAY

THURSDAY

FRIDAY

SATURDAY